THE ART
OF
OPTIMAL HEALTH

HOW TO ACHIEVE A LIFETIME OF RADIANT VITALITY

DR. CHAZ EBERT

ISBN-13: 978-1979927680
ISBN-10: 1979927685

SUCCESS STORIES

"We LOVE LOVE LOVE Dr. Ebert!" -Nikki

"My whole family is now truly healthy. Thank you, Dr. Ebert!" -M.H.

"I was curious at first, but Dr. Ebert has changed my life for the better…Thank you, Dr. Ebert!" -J.L.

"Wow!!! I wasn't sure what to expect, but I'm amazed at what I've learned. I love the way Dr. Ebert presents things - easy to understand and to the point. He even makes them fun while opening your eyes and mind to great wellness tips. I think this program is FANTASTIC!" -Christine V.

"Dr. Ebert was friendly and gave me so much information about what TRUE health is. I am so excited!" -M.M.

"Now, I'm living without daily pain, and rebuilding the strength and flexibility that I had lost!" -V.M.

"Dr. Ebert is very passionate about what he does. Loves to share his knowledge with you and ensures you fully understand it. Very friendly and a caring individual." -Wilson

"My experience with Dr. Ebert has been amazing. I feel much better. Just feel all around better. Trying to make healthier choices." -Joanna

"I'm able to enjoy my children a lot more, and I feel like a different person!" -Nicole D.

"Dr. Ebert has changed my life. I'm not in constant pain anymore, and I enjoy my life again!" -Cheryl W.

"Dr. Ebert has changed my life for the better!" -Allison J.

"What an amazing experience I have had with Dr. Ebert!" – Aaron B.

"My results have been amazing!! My husband, my daughter, and I are all enjoying the benefits of improved health." – Sandra B.

"I can't begin to say how much better I feel since working with Dr. Ebert!" – Harriett H.

DISCLAIMER:

PLEASE CONSULT WITH YOUR PHYSICIAN BEFORE STARTING ANY HEALTH, FITNESS, OR NUTRITION PROGRAM. THE USE OF ANY INFORMATION PROVIDED IN THIS BOOK IS SOLELY AT YOUR OWN RISK.

CONTENTS

INTRODUCTION

remember it like it was yesterday.

I was fresh out of school, and in a consultation with a sweet lady in her forties named Paula. During the consult, I discovered that Paula had been suffering a long time with, not only neck pain, back pain, and headaches, but also high blood pressure, diabetes, and weight management issues. Her whole life was affected by her health challenges: she couldn't exercise, she was missing days of work, she couldn't play with her kids, she was extremely stressed out, had no energy, and she was spending a large amount of money on her health concerns each and every month.

As we were finishing up the consult, Paula looked right at me, tears rolling down her face, and said, "I just don't want to die like my mom!"

As it turns out, Paula's mother had suffered with the same types of health challenges as Paula, and had died at a very early age. Paula was terrified that she was heading down the same road.

Have you ever had those moments in your life that just seem

to hit you right between the eyes and rattle your cage a bit? This was one of them for me!

I remember looking at Paula and saying, "You're in the right place! I'm confident that we can help you; and if you can stick to the game plan, your life will never be the same again!"

I also remember going home that night and thinking to myself, "I have to come up with a game plan for Paula that is going to work and get results!"

Then, I thought, "I wonder how many other people are out there suffering just like Paula? How could I help them?"

So I developed a simple, easy-to-follow, but effective game plan for Paula.

Fast forward a few short months, and Paula is a completely different person! She is pain-free, energetic, playing with her kids, and saving a ton of money each month!

Paula got her life back!

The health game plan that Paula followed is laid out for you in the pages of this book!

The game plan has morphed a bit since then, and will continue to change as newer and better health techniques come along. That being said, if you do the things contained in this book on a consistent basis, I'm confident you will be in the top 5% in the world when it comes to overall health.

Why listen to me?

I could bore you with doctorate degrees, credentials, and accomplishments, but who really cares about those things?

All I will tell you is that I have traveled hundreds of thousands of miles, spent hundreds of thousands of dollars, spent thousands of hours researching, studying, and learning the most advanced, natural health and wellness strategies in the world. I have been blessed to see these strategies get results in my own life, and in the lives of thousands of my patients! Results…isn't that what we really want?

A Few Things About This Book:

- My doctorate is NOT in English. Ha! My writing style is pretty laid back and conversational. Please forgive me for any grammatical errors. Thank you in advance!

- I hate "fluff"…especially in books. You know…the book that is 400+ pages that could have been 40 pages. I will get to the "X's and O's" of the health game plan as quickly as possible. I will give very brief reasons why I'm recommending something, but I will not bore you with all the research behind it. I encourage you to do your due diligence and perform your own research before incorporating anything into your health regime. Make sure they are actually respected and qualified resources. Also, when it comes to optimal health, I have found that simplicity is paramount!

- I have had many wonderful mentors, teachers, and coaches over the years. I want to give credit where credit is due. That being said, after studying optimal health and wellness for many years, it's actually quite difficult to determine where, when, and from whom I heard, read, or gathered information from. For example, I remember being blown away listening to Dr. James Chestnut talk about wellness (Eat Well, Move Well, Think Well), and incorporating this information into my life, but putting my own twist on things after tireless experimentation. My point is…I'd like to thank and give credit to all the people I have learned from, and in no way do I mean to take credit for any information that is not my own. I hope that makes sense.

How to Use This Book:

Listen, when it comes to health, there are thousands of "gurus" out there. It seems like there are about a million health tips that you need to do to be healthy. Not to mention, for every truly effective health tip, there is another "expert" telling you the exact opposite. That's just the way it is.

My goal is simplicity! I could give you a thousand things to do, but most people (not you, of course) won't take action because they are overwhelmed. When I am presenting health talks to groups or organizations, I try to minimize the action steps to 1-3 powerful things only!

That being said, I want you to get your money's worth from this book. So, we will be discussing the 5 key essentials to optimal health. Within those 5 essentials, I will give you the top 5 most powerful things you can do for each essential. These are the things that have gotten the best results for myself, my family, and my patients.

Can you do more? Of course! But I'm confident that if you ONLY did the things in this book, you'd be THRILLED with your state of health!

I challenge you to try and incorporate just one new health tip from each of the 5 essentials initially. That's it! Don't try to do all of them at once. If you implement just one health tip from each category, by the end of the month, you will be amazed at the positive shift in your health!

I have *starred* the health tip in each section that I believe is the most powerful (not always the easiest). Basically, if I could do only 1 of the 5 health tips in each section, I would do the *starred* tip.

Enough fluff…let's rock and roll!

HEALTH:
YOUR #1 GREATEST ASSET

"When you have your health, you have every-thing! When you do not have your health, nothing else matters at all!"– Austin Burroughs

Think about it…if you don't have your health, it doesn't really matter how much money you make, how big your home is, how nice your car is. Everything in your life revolves around your health: your relationships, your finances, your emotions, your physical activities, and even your spiritual purpose in life.

So, if health is our #1 greatest asset, why do we take it for granted? Why do we ignore and neglect it? Why don't we protect it? Why don't we invest in it?

I believe optimal health equals ultimate freedom. When you have your health (i.e. vitality, energy, and mobility), you have the freedom to do the things you love to do: travel, play golf, exercise, perform your job effectively, play with your kids or grandkids, be a wonderful spouse! Most importantly, your focus can be on a purpose bigger than yourself by serving others.

When you don't have your health (i.e. sickness, disease, pain), you're not able to do the things you love to do…or at least not as well. Most importantly, and understandably, your focus turns within, and you're unable to serve others effectively.

The Dalai Lama sums it all up. When asked what surprises him the most, he offered this insightful response:

"Man. Because he sacrifices his health in order to make money. Then he sacrifices money to recuperate his health. And then he is so anxious about the future that he does not enjoy the present; the result being that he does not live in the present or the future; he lives as if he is never going to die, and then dies having never really lived."

My hope for you, with this book, is that you come away with a game plan to help you avoid sickness, disease, pain, unnecessary drugs, unnecessary surgeries, and live a life full of health and radiant vitality!

So, I'm going to start out with the most important health tip you'll ever need…and it's in the form of a question:

WHY do you want to be healthy?

Take your time before you answer this!

If you can truly answer that question, the rest will just fall into place!

You see, I can give you all the best health tips and tell you exactly WHAT to do. But if you don't have a good enough reason WHY, you won't take action or stay disciplined to see the results you desire.

Once you come up with your answer, I'm going to challenge you to ask yourself WHY 6 more times (7 total). Not 8; 7 times total! Then you will have your true WHY…your true purpose! (Don't be surprised if this exercise becomes very emotional for you…it's supposed to!)

Let me give you an example of what this could look like:

1. WHY do I want to be healthy?

   o   I want to have more energy!

2. WHY?

   o   If I had more energy, I could be more productive!

3. WHY?

   o   If I was more productive, I would be more valuable at my job!

4. WHY?

   o   If I was more valuable at my job, I could get a raise and earn more money!

5. WHY?

   o   If I could earn more money, I could support my family better!

6. WHY?

   o   If I could support my family better, my children would have better opportunities in life!

7. WHY?

   o   If my children have better opportunities, I will feel fulfilled as a person and as a parent!

Powerful stuff! Would you agree?

I encourage you to write down your final answer…your BIG WHY…your true purpose for being healthy, and put it in a place where you'll see it every day!

It will be the motivation you need to stay strong and reach your goals!

Now that you have your WHY, it's time to take some action!

EAT WELL

If you have an apple or a donut, which one is healthier? You got it (apple fritters, while delicious, don't count)!

The point is, you're smart! For the most part, we all know what we should be putting in our bodies and what we shouldn't. But yet, many of us (myself included) struggle with our diet and nutrition from time to time.

Let's change that!

* Intermittent Fasting

Just imagine never having to count calories again! I have used Intermittent Fasting (IF) for the past 8 years, and it has made a HUGE difference in my life. Intermittent Fasting is simply an eating pattern that cycles between periods of eating and fasting, and has been shown to:

- Decrease risk of cancer

- Decrease inflammation

- Improve cell function

- Help lose weight

- Decrease risk of diabetes

- Improve heart health

- Help cells repair

- Improve brain function

- Decrease risk of Alzheimer's

- Extend your lifespan

There are several methods of Intermittent Fasting, but I will discuss the two most popular:

- Eat Stop Eat: involves fasting for 24 hours (from dinner to dinner) one or two days a week. You are still eating every day, but you are basically skipping breakfast and lunch on your fasting days.

- 16/8 Method: involves eating your meals within an 8-hour window each day, and fasting for the remaining 16 hours. This is the method I use, and I find it easy (after the first couple of weeks). You can pick whatever 8-hour window you want, but my window is 12 – 8 PM, which simply means that I don't eat anything for breakfast or after dinner. You can basically eat as many meals as you want within your 8-hour window. Obviously, the healthier items you eat, the better your health will become! Also, you can, and should, still drink water during your fasting window.

Please note, fasting is contraindicated for several conditions, including:

- Malignant arrhythmia

- Protein wasting disease (e.g. lupus, Cushing's syndrome)

- Major system failure (e.g. liver failure, renal failure)

- Drug therapy causing protein wasting (steroids, anti-neoplastic agents)

- Metastatic cancer (stage IV)

- Diabetes, type 1, juvenile

- Severe osteoporosis

- MI or stroke within the last 6 months

- Anorexia or Body Mass Index (BMI) less than 18.5

- Pregnancy or lactation

Please consult your physician before trying Intermittent Fasting.

FRESH FIBER FIRST

Before each meal, even if it's going to be a meal full of Big Macs and donuts, try to eat some raw, fresh fruits or vegetables first. It can be anything you like: salad, celery, carrots, strawberries, blueberries, etc.

Not only will you get great nutrients from these things, but also, they will trigger the release of enzymes in your body that will make you feel fuller, faster. This will help you eat less "junk" on the back end of your meals. Think about it… have you ever eaten your way through a whole bag of potato chips? I know I have. What about a whole bag of celery? Probably not. Your body just says, "I'm good. That's enough." That's the power of Fresh Fiber First.

HARA HACHI BU

Hara what??? This is an old Japanese saying that basically means 'stop eating when you're 80% full.' Why? Neurologically, it takes about 20 minutes for the brain to realize that the stomach is full. When you're 80% full, you're actually full, but your brain just doesn't know it yet. Have you ever said to yourself, "You know what, I think I'll do one more piece of pizza (or one more pancake)," and then 20 minutes later, you felt like you were going to explode! Yeah…same here!

By practicing Hara Hachi Bu, the Okinawans have become some of the healthiest, longest living people in the world!

DECREASE SUGAR

This one sounds simple, but might be the most difficult to implement. Sugar is in just about everything!

We have all been affected by cancer in some way. I realize there are many different forms of cancer, but here's the thing… cancer cells LOVE sugar! Cancer feeds on sugar!

The first thing we need to do is start limiting sugar intake from sweets, candy, soda, white bread, even pasta and dairy milk. So much easier said than done!

If you're looking at labels, anything that ends in "-ose" is sugar.

Now, whenever you cut something negative out of your life, you have to replace it with something positive. I highly recommend you start adding in healthy fats such as avocados, nuts, seeds, healthy butter, coconut oil, extra virgin olive oil, wild-caught salmon, and grass-fed beef.

Many people have had life-changing results using a Ketogenic Diet (5% carbs, 25% protein, 75% healthy fats). I highly recommend you look into this type of diet, as it has shown to help with weight loss, reduce the risk of type II diabetes, reduce the risk of heart disease, reduce the risk of cancer, fight brain disease, and increase longevity.

SUPPLEMENTS

Every day, I'm asked, "Doc, what supplements should I be taking?"

This is a tough question because everybody is unique and different.

First of all, the goal is to get your nutrients mostly from a healthy diet. That being said, the truth is, our soils have become depleted of essential nutrients needed for optimal health.

Due to these major deficiencies in our soil and diets, I want to discuss the supplements that I believe virtually everyone should be taking every day.

If you go to your local health store, there are literally thousands of supplements on the shelves that you could take.

All supplements should be 100% certified organic and synthetic-free. Let's face it, you get what you pay for. If you get the "bottom-shelf" supplements, there is a very good chance that absorption of the nutrients will be very low. Essentially, you'll have very expensive urine!

If you could only take four supplements, these would be the four I would recommend:

Multi-Vitamin: the benefits of a multi-vitamin supplement are boosted energy, increased longevity, enhanced weight loss, and improved nervous system function.

Omega-3: the benefits of an omega-3 supplement are increased heart health, increased brain health, cancer prevention, and inflammation reduction.

Probiotic: the benefits of a probiotic supplement are improved digestive function, boosted immune system, reduced acid reflux, and increased mental health.

Vitamin D: the benefits of a vitamin D supplement are increased immune function, decreased risk of heart disease, decreased risk of cancer, and reduced inflammation.

A few "Honorable Mention" supplements that have helped me, and I believe would help most people would include:

Vitamin B Complex: increases energy, nervous system function, and immune system function.

Antioxidant: reduces inflammation by protecting the body from free radical damage.

Magnesium: a natural muscle relaxer that helps with digestion, cramps, and even headaches.

Turmeric: a powerful spice that has been shown to decrease inflammation, improve brain function, help depression, improve heart health, combat arthritis, and even help kill cancer cells.

Overall, the best and simplest diet advice I've ever heard comes from Michael Pollen. It's a 7-word diet:

Eat food. Mostly plants. Not too much.

Meaning…eat real food (not synthetic, processed, man-made junk). The majority of your diet should be plant-based, and stop eating when you're 80% full.

Simple, right? You've got this!

MOVE WELL

Our bodies were made to move! Unfortunately, in today's society, we do a lot of sitting, don't we? Sitting is the new smoking, but motion is medicine!

The #1 killer in the United States is heart disease. Research shows that consistent exercise can reduce your risk of heart disease by up to 50%. Those are some great numbers in your favor! So get moving!

TOP 5 HEALTH TIPS:
MOVE WELL

* HIGH-INTENSITY INTERVAL TRAINING (HIIT)

One of the things I always hear is, "Doc, I just don't have the time to work out!"

I realize we're all busy these days. It makes me cringe when

I see people trying to lose weight by spending hours upon hours on the treadmill, elliptical, exercise bike, running, or any other type of long, slow, boring cardio. If you enjoy it… great! But it might not be the most effective way to get great results.

The most recent research shows that short, intense workouts/cardio burn more fat and build more muscle than long, slow, boring workouts/cardio. One study showed that just 60 seconds worth of max effort "bursts" can burn fat for up to 38 hours afterward! 60 seconds of work…38 hours of fat burning. Not a bad return on your investment of time, huh?

Human growth hormone, a hormone responsible for burning fat and building muscle, is released based on intensity, not duration.

It is critical that you consult with your physician before attempting HIIT!

Here's the beautiful thing…you need very little, if any, equipment. You don't need a gym membership. Heck, you can do this in your pajamas in a hotel room if needed (don't laugh…I've done it many times!)

You can simply march, jog, or run in place as fast as you can.

The key is to go all out, max effort. Everybody's max effort is different, and that's why this type of work out is scalable for anybody. For example, your max effort might just be marching in place. That's great! You might be able to jog in place. Awesome! Or, you might be in pretty good shape and be able to sprint with high knees. Fantastic!

You can also use many other methods: jumping jacks, burpees, jump rope, elliptical, spin bike, kettlebell swings, line jumps, treadmill sprints, etc.

There are many effective work-to-rest ratios when it comes

to HIIT (AKA Burst Training). My favorite is 20 seconds of work, followed by 10-60 seconds of rest. I prefer the number of "bursts" to range from 3 to 8. You may just want to start with 1 burst and build from there.

You can alter the difficulty by adding bursts, decreasing rest, or both.

For example, my "Go To" burst training when I'm short on time is 3 x 20/20. Meaning 3 "bursts" lasting 20 seconds, followed by 20 seconds of rest between each burst. I'll run in place as fast as I can for 20 seconds, rest for 20 seconds, and repeat 2 more times for a total of 3 bursts. Done in a total of 2 minutes! Amazing!

To keep things fresh, sometimes I'll do 8 x 20/60 (8 bursts x 20-second burst / 60 seconds rest between bursts). Other times, I'll do what's known as Tabata Training: 8 x 20/10. 8 bursts total, 20-second bursts, only 10 seconds rest between bursts. I would NOT recommend this for most people! It is INTENSE!!! I simply want to give you ways of altering the difficulty and keeping things fresh by using different exercises and work/rest ratios.

Just imagine all the time you'll save, the great results you'll notice, and wear and tear you'll prevent on all your joints.

WALKING

I am a HUGE proponent of walking! I truly believe it is the best thing we can do for not only our bodies but our minds and nervous systems. Walking creates motion in many joints of the body, and motion is medicine. It also "reboots" the nervous system, helping your body function at its best. Walking is also a weight-bearing exercise that builds and protects bone density while avoiding the damage done to the spine and joints by other exercises. Also, some studies have shown walking to be just as effective as antidepressant medication. I believe walking/exercise is the most potent and underutilized antidepressant in the world…and it's free!

Research also shows that walking 140-175 minutes per week (20-25 minutes per day) adds anywhere from 3-7 years to an individual's lifespan.

Try going for a brisk walk. Shoot for 20 minutes (about a mile, give or take). Do that every day for a few weeks and notice how you feel and function (both mind and body). If you'd like, you can extend your walks up to 60+ minutes, increase your pace, or both. As far as pace, think about how you would walk in the airport if you were trying to catch a flight, but it took a little longer than expected to get through security (I'm guessing you know exactly what I'm talking about).

Also, think about our ancestors, the hunters, and gatherers. They didn't do moderate intensity, long, slow, boring cardio. They walked and roamed until it was time to hunt, and then they sprinted! What a perfect combination! They were lean, fit, healthy, and I'd bet anything, they had a fraction of the heart disease or diabetes that the current population experiences (if it could've somehow been tested back then).

For a perfect combo workout of HIIT and walking, perform a 3 x 20/20 burst workout (2 minutes), then go for a 20-minute brisk walk. 22 minutes total! Be sure to do the burst training BEFORE walking, as it will increase fat burning.

YOGA

The benefits of yoga have been well researched. They include:

- Increased strength
- Increased flexibility
- Decreased stress

- Decreased neck & back pain
- Improved spinal health
- Improved weight control

Those are just a few benefits. There are many more. I repeat, motion is medicine. By continually moving your joints and spine, you keep them from locking up, wearing down, and forming arthritis. Also, PM yoga (done in the evening) can help you relax, unwind, and get much better, deeper sleep!

Don't be fooled. Yoga is not just laid-back stretching. It can be quite the challenge. You will be using muscles you don't typically use, in positions you're typically not in on a regular basis. Yoga does a wonderful job of counteracting many problems caused by the amount of sitting we do these days.

I highly encourage you to visit your local yoga studio and try out a class. If you're new to yoga, and that sounds intimidating, don't panic. There are thousands of awesome yoga videos online for free! You can try yoga in the privacy of your own home.

One caution: be sure you have no spinal or joint contraindications for yoga or certain poses. While yoga is generally safe, I have seen people injure themselves performing certain poses that are not right for their spine and bodies. As with anything, just be careful. If something doesn't feel right, stop.

STRENGTH TRAINING: SUPER SLOW REPETITION & RESISTANCE BAND TRAINING

SUPER SLOW REPETITION TRAINING:

When it comes to strength training, there are three types of workouts that I prefer: super slow repetition, resistance band, and bodyweight training.

In this section, we'll discuss Super Slow Rep and Resistance Band training (Bodyweight training will be discussed in the next section).

In addition to core and cardio/interval training, any strength training regimen should include the following 3 types of exercises:

1. Squatting Movement (i.e. squats, lunges)

2. Pushing Movement (i.e. chest press, military press)

3. Pulling Movement (i.e. row, pulldown)

Super Slow Repetition training consists of performing only one set of each exercise to failure (unable to perform another rep), but performing the exercise as slowly as possible, and using a weight/resistance that causes you to reach failure between 8-12 reps, increasing weight/resistance once you surpass 12 reps.

You can use free weights for Super Slow Rep training, but I actually prefer using machines to help prevent injury (especially if you don't have a spotter, which is always recommended).

Let's take a machine chest press, for example. You would choose a weight that you think would cause you to reach failure between 8-12 reps (it might take a few times to get the resistance correct). You would then perform a chest press, moving the weight as slowly as possible during the entire movement. Each repetition should take about 20 seconds (10 seconds of pushing, 10 seconds of lowering the weight back to starting position). There should be no stopping/resting at the "top" or "bottom" of the lift, and no momentum used to start the lift. Think of it as one big, long, slow repetition instead of 8-12 separate reps. If you can perform more than 12 reps, use a heavier weight next time. If you perform less than 8 reps, use a lighter weight next time.

You can use the same Super Slow Rep concept with exercises like machine leg press (be sure to keep the arch in your lower back while performing leg press to prevent damaging lumbar discs) and the machine row.

So, an example of a 20-minute Super Slow Rep Workout might look something like this:

1. Warm-Up (5 mins): dynamic bodyweight warm-up or bike/elliptical

2. Machine Leg Press (8-12 Super Slow Reps)

3. Machine Chest Press (8-12 Super Slow Reps)

4. Machine Row (8-12 Super Slow Reps)

5. Core (60 sec each): left plank, right plank, front plank

6. Cardio/HIIT (3x 20 sec ON/20 sec OFF = 2 mins): high knees

You'll love how these workouts are very short but extremely challenging and effective.

RESISTANCE BAND TRAINING:

For resistance band training, you could use the same workout described above, but substitute resistance band exercises instead of the Super Slow Rep exercises.

I'm confident you will grow to love using resistance bands for your strength training. They are easy on the joints, keep the muscles pliable, and you can use them anywhere, especially when traveling.

With resistance bands, I recommend performing as many quality, high-paced reps as possible within three, 20-second sets, with 20 seconds of rest between sets. Similar to the 3 x 20/20 Burst Training described earlier, but with resistance exercises instead of cardio exercises.

An example of a resistance band training workout might look something like this:

RB = Resistance Band
AMRAP = As Many Reps As Possible

1. Warm-Up (5 mins): dynamic bodyweight warm-up or bike/elliptical

2. RB Squat (AMRAP; 3 x 20 sec ON/20 sec OFF)

3. RB Chest Press (AMRAP; 3 x 20 sec ON/20 sec OFF)

4. RB Row (AMRAP; 3 x 20 sec ON/20 sec OFF)

5. Core (60 sec each): cat/cow, curl up, right plank, left plank, bird dog

6. Cardio/HIIT (3 x 20 sec ON/20 sec OFF = 2 mins): elliptical sprints

That's it...simple!

Big 6 Bodyweight Workout

If I could perform and/or recommend only one workout, it would be the Big 6 Bodyweight Workout. It combines strength training, core training, and cardio training all within a 3-12 minute workout, and with virtually no equipment required.

It is a workout that includes the following 6 bodyweight (BW) exercises:

1. BW Squats

2. Push Ups

3. Stick-Ups (or Band Pulls)

4. BW Reverse Lunges

5. Cross-Body Mountain Climbers (or Front Plank)

6. Sprint in Place

*If you are unfamiliar with an exercise, a simple search on Google or YouTube will help you find articles/videos on how to perform each movement.

You will do each of the 6 bodyweight exercises for 30 seconds, performing as many reps as possible for each exercise. That's one circuit, which will take you just 3 minutes. You can perform 1-3 circuits, with 0-60 seconds rest between circuits. You can increase or decrease the intensity by manipulating the number of reps performed, the number of circuits performed, and/or the amount of rest between circuits.

1 Circuit / 60 Seconds Rest = Beginner

2 Circuits / 30 Seconds Rest = Intermediate

3 Circuits / 0 Seconds Rest = Advanced

The majority of the time I will perform 2 circuits with no rest between circuits, and be done in 6 minutes. Do not be fooled by the fact that this workout is short. It is intense, and an excellent way to burn fat and build muscle in minimal time. It can also be done just about anywhere, making it the perfect workout for busy moms and dads, or the traveling business person.

Remember, motion is medicine. Our bodies were meant to move. The best way to get in shape is to never get out of it!

THINK WELL

et me ask you…any stress in your life? That's what I thought!
As stated earlier, the #1 killer in the United States is heart disease. What do you think is one of the leading causes of heart disease? You got it…stress!

We all have stress. It could be financial stress, relationship stress, job stress, etc.

Stress can wreak havoc on your health by affecting the way your nervous system functions, leading to a decreased performance of your organs, tissues, and cells.

Here's a little secret…stress is not going away! We're always going to have bills to pay, deadlines, and obligations that will lead to stress.

The key is, we must do things to counteract stress so that it doesn't affect our health!

* MEDITATION

One of the most powerful things I have ever done for my health has been meditating on a daily basis. For over the past year and a half, I have meditated every day for 10 minutes. You can meditate for as short or as long as you want. Many people recommend 20-minute meditations twice per day (morning and evening), but even 1-minute meditations are powerful. For me, one daily 10-minute meditation works great! I've noticed it helps me with my focus, energy, attitude, stress, weight, and overall health. Research supports these benefits as well.

Now listen, you do not need to become a monk, a hippie, or burn incense to start meditating.

The most basic description of meditation I've ever heard is that you simply focus on an "anchor" for a certain time. Not an actual anchor that you drop out of your boat, but rather something that you will direct all your attention to during your meditation time. An anchor could be your breathing, a word, a phrase/mantra, a sound, a body part, or just about anything that is productive for you!

The two anchors that I use the most would be:

- Breathing: focusing on inhaling through my nose while my belly expands, and exhaling through my mouth while my belly lowers

- Phrase/Mantra: repeating a phrase or mantra silently

to myself over and over. Examples: "I love myself"/"I am confident"/"Peace"/"Release"

If you're a beginner, you'll soon realize how difficult it is to stay focused on your anchor for even just a few minutes. Your mind will start to wander to other thoughts. Perfectly normal. Don't get frustrated! Once you realize that your focus has drifted, simply let those thoughts go, and calmly return your focus to your anchor. After a while, you will notice your mind wandering less and less, and your focus on your anchor becoming stronger and stronger.

So, here's what to do:

1. Try to find a quiet, peaceful spot

2. Set a timer (as much time as you want...I recommend 10-20 minutes)

3. Choose your anchor (i.e. breathing or phrase/mantra)

4. Start timer

5. Focus on anchor until timer goes off (If your mind wanders, simply release the thought, and return your focus to your anchor)

That's it. That's meditation! It's very simple, but extremely powerful!

If you need a little help getting started, I highly recommend you find a guided meditation online that you can follow. I also recommend an app called Headspace that you can download on your phone that will guide you through daily 10-minute meditations. Another excellent meditation resource is a book called *Love Yourself Like Your Life Depends On It* by Kamal Ravikant. It's a crazy title with a crazy cover, but it is one of the most powerful books I've ever read!

Another great technique is called 4-7-8 Breathing. Hence the name, it is a powerful breathing technique that decreases anxiety, lowers blood pressure, and helps you get to sleep quickly.

Here's what to do:

1. Inhale through your nose for a count of 4

2. Hold your breath for a count of 7

3. Exhale through your mouth for a count of 8

*Perform 4-8 breathes. Do this at least twice daily.

This will only take you a couple of minutes. But if you do this on a regular basis, after about 8 weeks, you should notice that you are calmer, more relaxed, and get to sleep MUCH quicker. There are times that I put my head on the pillow at night, start 4-7-8 breathing, and the next thing I know my alarm is going off the next morning. Powerful stuff!

SLEEP

The quality and quantity of your sleep have a MAJOR effect on your health. The vast majority of all your body's healing, repairing, and regenerating happens while you are asleep. So, if you're not getting enough quality sleep, all of your organs, tissues, and cells will continue to break down, leading to sickness and disease.

The average adult requires 7-9 hours of quality, uninterrupted sleep.

Besides the 4-7-8 breathing technique described earlier, another powerful technique for restful sleep is the 10-3-2-1-0 Rule. Here's how it goes:

10 – No caffeine within 10 hours of bedtime

3 – No food or alcohol within 3 hours of bedtime

2 – No work-related activities within 2 hours of bedtime

1 – No electronics (TV, phone, iPad) within 1 hour of bedtime

0 – The number of times you will hit the SNOOZE button in the morning

A FEW OTHER SLEEP TIPS INCLUDE:

- Keep room dark and cool (60-67 degrees)

- Sleep on back or side (left side if you suffer with acid reflux)

- Invest in a quality mattress and pillow (as firm as you can handle)

- Remove electronics from bedroom (i.e. cell phones, TV, computers)

- Keep bedroom clean (consider an air purifier, dehumidifier, and/or plant)

- Use a sound machine

- Consider placing a pillow under or between your knees

- Exercise (preferably in the morning)

- Write out your next day's To-Do List before bed (allows mind to relax)

- Take a warm bath or shower before bed

- Chiropractic care helps sleep tremendously

- Perform PM yoga before bed

- Write in a "Gratitude Journal" each night

- Pray / Meditate

- Read a fictional book

- Use a mask and/or earplugs

- Try to be asleep by 10:30 PM

- Try to have a consistent bedtime and wake time

NEUROPLASTICITY

Neuroplasticity: the ability of your brain to reorganize itself, both physically and functionally, throughout your life due to your environment, behavior, thinking, and emotions.

Your brain is just like a muscle. It can adapt and change throughout your lifetime (in a positive or negative way). For your brain to function properly, you must train it on a regular basis for positive changes. Think of it as brain fitness. We work our muscles through strength training and stretching, but rarely do we spend dedicated time training our brain. Like the old saying goes... use it or lose it!

I truly believe that proper "brain training" is a major key to preventing/helping certain neurodegenerative and psychological diseases such as Alzheimer's disease, Parkinson's disease, PTSD, ADD, ADHD, depression, and traumatic brain injuries.

Training your brain for increased neuroplasticity is actually a lot easier, and more fun, than you might think! Basically, by thinking, solving problem, or learning, you are increasing neuroplasticity.

There are several apps/websites that will take you through different types of brain training. One app/website that I recommend is called BrainHQ. They have trainings that test your memory, decision-making, cognition, and attention.

There are also many simple ways to get your brain training:

- Learning a foreign language

- Learning a new instrument

- Crossword puzzles

- Sudoku

- Reading

- Traveling

- Using your non-dominant hand for tasks (i.e. brushing your teeth)

- Dancing

- Painting / Drawing

- Meditation

- Getting enough sleep

- Learning how to use new technology (i.e. smartphone or tablet)

These are just a few examples. But like I said, brain training can actually be pretty fun! Anything that forces your brain to get out of auto-pilot mode and do something new is increasing neuroplasticity and protecting your brain from degeneration!

I'm confident that you will notice a big improvement in your social and professional life if you commit to the proper brain training!

THE 3 G'S (GROWTH, GIVING, & GRATITUDE)

GROWTH:

One of the biggest keys to success, happiness, and fulfillment in life is PROGRESS! Progress equals growth…growth equals feeling alive! If you're not growing, you're dying.

Think about it…whether it be weight loss, finances, or your golf game, if you're making progress, even small/slow progress, you feel motivated to continue to work toward your goals. It's when progress halts, we hit a plateau, or start heading backward when depression and negative thinking creep in.

Done is better than perfect! Start today…anything! Just start!

If it's weight loss, start with a short walk. If it's lowering your golf handicap, go hit a few putts. If you want to become an expert on a topic, pick up a book and start reading a few pages. START!!!

With every decision you make, it will either lead you toward your goal or away from it. Just keep moving in the right direction and be patient. As long as you keep making progress, you can't lose!

I challenge you to spend at least 15 minutes per day doing something to help you grow in the desired area of your life. For example, read a book, listen to a podcast, or watch a video on YouTube that will help develop the skills you need to grow and advance in the area you have chosen. After just one year, you will have spent 91.25 hours on that subject. I promise that you will experience growth in this area of your life!

GIVING:

> *"We make a living by what we get; we make a life by what we give."- Winston Churchill*

> *"For it is in giving that we receive."- Saint Francis of Assisi*

> *"The secret to living is giving!"- Tony Robbins*

Many studies have shown that we are happier and more fulfilled when we give rather than receive. Call it karma, or whatever you want, but there seems to be a universal law that when we give, we receive regardless. It's so easy to become focused on ourselves rather than serving others. Trust me, I'm as guilty as anybody. If we can somehow get outside our own little bubble, and seek opportunities to give and serve others, we will truly be happy and fulfilled. We need to shift our focus from what we're not getting to what we can give! How can you add more value to other people's lives? There are many ways to give: money, time, knowledge, expertise, advice, volunteering, coaching, etc.

We all have strengths or expertise. Take some time to determine your strengths, think about people who could benefit from your strengths, then go serve these people with your strengths!

Also, we all have hard times now and again, but there is ALWAYS somebody worse off than yourself. I challenge you to find somebody that you can mentor. Somebody who would give anything to be in your shoes (even in your hard times). Connect with them. Help them. Lift them up. Watch how it affects YOUR life! It's a win-win!

A mentor of mine told me that whatever you want more of… give more of! If you want more money, give more money! If you want more love, give more love! If you want more help, give more help! You get the idea...let's make it happen!

GRATITUDE:

I know it's cliché, but developing an "attitude of gratitude" is critical to living a fulfilled life.

You could seemingly have it all (money, cars, houses, toys, fame), but if you're not grateful for those things, they will never be enough. Unfortunately, many celebrities have found this out the hard way.

It's so easy to think of all the things we don't have and stress about how we're going to acquire them. However, if you can simply take time to recognize all the blessings in your life that you currently do have, it completely shifts your mental and physiological state.

How many times throughout your day does "not enough" cross your mind?

- I didn't get enough sleep.

- We don't have enough money.

- I don't have enough time.

- I didn't get enough done today.

If we're not careful, we can find ourselves in a constant mindset of scarcity. This scarcity mindset leads to fear and anger, which are two of the biggest hurdles to living a happy and fulfilled life.

Here's the good news...your brain can only focus on one thing at a time. It is literally impossible to be grateful and fearful at the same time. It is literally impossible to be grateful and angry at the same time. So, the choice is yours...yes, it is a choice! Choose gratitude or fear? Gratitude or anger? Choose to be grateful, even on your worst day, and decide that you will focus on gratitude!

Also, gratitude plays a key role in your success in sports, health, business, and other areas of life. You can literally program your nervous system for success through gratitude. Let me ask you, when was the last time you celebrated? I'm not talking about birthdays or holidays (those are great), but rather when you set a goal, achieved the goal, and truly rewarded yourself? Can you recall? What typically happens is, we set a goal, determine a reward for reaching the goal, hit our goal, and then say to ourselves, "Ahh…I don't really need that reward, and it's a little expensive…I'm good…. What's next?" FAIL!!! When we do this, we program our nervous system for failure, not success. What if you had a boss that said, "Alright gang, if we hit this revenue goal by the end of the quarter, everybody will receive a $10,000 bonus!" So, you work your butt off to reach the revenue goal and succeed! Your boss comes in the next day and says, "Great job gang! You did it… you hit the goal! Unfortunately, you will NOT be receiving the $10,000 bonus that we talked about. Sorry!" How would you respond? How would that make you feel? Would you ever again work hard for that boss to reach another goal? Hell no! But that's what we do to ourselves all the time!

Here's my point…if you set a goal (even a small goal), determine a reward, and hit your goal… CELEBRATE!!! You EARNED it! Take it all in too… the whole process of the reward! Your reward should be relative to your goal. It might be buying yourself a new shirt when you lose some weight, or it might be a week-long vacation to Hawaii when you earn a promotion. Take it all in… trying the new shirt on and feeling how good you look, or feeling the sun on your skin while you lay on the beach! Incorporate and remember as many senses as you can while experiencing your reward process.

Be grateful for the reward that you earned! By rewarding yourself, you will program your nervous system for success!

Gratitude acts like a magnet. It attracts more of what you're grateful for. Just like we discussed about giving, if you want more of something, be grateful for it. If you want more money, be grateful for the money you have. If you want more clients, be grateful for the clients you have. If you want more love, be grateful for the love you have. If you want more health, be grateful for the health you have.

One of the most powerful things you can do is start a Gratitude Journal. Very simply, leave a notebook and pen on your bedside table, and every night before you go to sleep, write down three things you were grateful for that day. It could be anything you were grateful for throughout the day. Heck, if you had a rough day, it might be, "I'm grateful that the dog took a crap on the tile versus the carpet!" Ha! Be sure to write down at least three things. Then, leave your Gratitude Journal on your bedside table so that it's the first thing you see when you wake up. What a great way to start your day!!! Your Gratitude Journal will allow you to "bookend" your day with gratitude instead of fear or anger!

DAILY RITUALS

Discipline creates freedom! Most people shy away from discipline, order, routine, or accountability because they feel it will confine or limit them. Nothing could be further from the truth. When we develop powerful daily rituals that set us up for success, we create the abundance of freedom that everyone is chasing these days.

How do we do that? I recommend you spend some time each morning and evening in four quadrants of personal development: spiritual, mental, emotional, and physical. How much time you spend in each quadrant is completely up to you.

You could spend 15 minutes in each quadrant, and you have your own Hour of Power. You could spend 2 minutes in each quadrant, and you have your own Great in 8. The important part is that you spend some time in these quadrants each day, ideally in the morning and evening (Exception: unless it's PM yoga or something calming, avoid exercising within 3 hours of bedtime, as it can affect your sleep).

You can do whatever you want, but here are some ideas for each quadrant to get you started:

SPIRITUAL:

- Praying
- Reading the Bible or a devotional
- Listening to a message/sermon
- Watching a message/sermon

MENTAL:

- Reading a self-development/skill/professional book
- Listening to a self-development/skill/professional audio
- Watching a self-development/skill/professional video
- Brain Training

EMOTIONAL:

- Meditation
- 4-7-8 Breathing

- Affirmations

- Gratitude Journal

PHYSICAL:

- Burst Training (HIIT)

- Walking

- Yoga

- Resistance Band, Super Slow Rep, or Big 6 Bodyweight Workout

You will be amazed at how your energy, attitude, and productivity will increase when you start implementing daily rituals to help you win the day!

Remember, we can choose what we focus on. I challenge you to choose a positive, happy, grateful mindset!

MINIMIZE TOXINS

Much like stress, we'll never be able to avoid 100% of toxins. They're in the air we breathe, medications, what we eat, what we drink...everywhere!

We can, however, do some things to limit our exposure to toxins and eliminate toxins from our body to prevent their harmful effects on our health!

* HYDRATION

One of the easiest and best ways to detoxify and help your body function optimally is to drink plenty of water. Roughly, 70% of our bodies are made up of water. Water helps flush the lymphatic system of toxins that we all acquire in everyday life.

I always get asked how much water is enough. Well, body types are different. To say everybody should drink 8 cups of water per day is ridiculous. Your goal should be to shoot for ½ your body weight in ounces of quality water each day. For example, if you way 160 lbs., you're shooting for 80 ounces of water every day. I know that sounds like a lot, but if you can do it, you will notice a huge difference in your energy levels, the way your muscles feel, the way your joints feel, the way your skin looks, and even improvement in digestion. Feel free to add a fresh lemon or electrolytes to your water to improve flavor and help decrease inflammation in your body.

You want to spread out your water intake throughout the day, but I highly recommend drinking a large glass of water first thing in the morning, as your body is dehydrated from still functioning throughout the night while you're sleeping. One thing, try to limit drinking water during meals, as it will interfere with digestion. Wait about an hour after your meal to continue your water intake.

Also, for every soda, coffee, or alcoholic beverage (which dehydrate you), you need to add 8 ounces of water. So, if you weight 200 lbs., and drink 2 cups of coffee, your goal is to drink 116 ounces of water during the day. You can do it!

Now, there are many different types of water. I recommend avoiding tap water (polluted with agricultural runoff, chemicals, chlorine, and prescription drugs), and shoot for drinking purified water or filtered water through a home filtration unit or oxidizing system.

NATURAL / ORGANIC FOOD & PRODUCTS

Try to eat and use the most natural/organic food and products. Yes, it might be a little more expensive, but it is an investment in your health. Trust me, it's much cheaper than drugs, surgeries, sickness, and disease from loading your body up with toxins from synthetic, chemical-filled food and products. Be careful of labels or advertising that says "Natural" or "Organic," as they might not be. A good rule of thumb is to look at the ingredients label. If there are ingredients that a 3rd grader couldn't pronounce, you probably shouldn't be putting that item in or on your body.

As for food, you should be eating things that were alive at one point (i.e. plants, animals) and will eventually rot within a short time (unlike packaged products, such as Twinkies, that last forever).

As for household products, skin care, etc., check out EWG. org. They rate products on how natural and safe they are. It is a great resource for many different products.

CLEANSE / DETOX

I'm a big proponent of periodic, natural cleanses or detoxifications. Even if you're doing a great job limiting toxins in your diet and household products, you will still acquire toxins. A cleanse or detoxification process can help clear your body of these toxins. There are many different cleanse/detox products out there. You will have to do your due diligence and determine what will be best for you. Personally, I have been very pleased with a product called Detoxx from Organixx (Just FYI…I get nothing in return for recommending these products).

There are many benefits of detoxification. They include:

- Weight Loss

- Increased Energy

- Decreased Headaches

- Improved Digestion

- Controlled Cravings

- Boosted Immune System

- Clearer Thinking

- Clearer Skin

- Better Breath

You see, most toxins in the body are absorbed by fat. So, the more toxic you are, the more fat your body has to hold onto in order to absorb the toxins. Guess what happens when you get rid of the toxins? You got it… Your body now doesn't need all the fat to absorb the toxins, and you should notice some weight/fat loss.

As always, please discuss your health situation with your doctor before attempting a cleanse/detox, especially if taking medications, pregnant, or breastfeeding.

SWEAT

Another simple, natural, and effective way to detoxify is to sweat. Your skin is your largest organ, and it plays a huge role in preventing toxins from getting into your body, and also moving toxins out. When you sweat, your pores open up, allowing toxins to move out of your body.

Sweating helps your body:

- Detoxify

- Maintain proper body temperature

- Improve acne and skin conditions

- Improver circulation

- Relieve stress / Improve relaxation

- Kill viruses and bacteria

The simplest way to sweat is by exercising (see previous Move Well chapter). Rebounding, or bouncing on a mini trampoline, is a very effective way to sweat and flush toxins out of your lymphatic system.

Another powerful way to sweat is by using a sauna, specifically a far-infrared sauna that heats you from the inside-out, accelerating and improving detoxification.

A simple rule is to sweat every day. It will help your body detoxify and function optimally!

TOXICITY / DEFICIENCY

This health tip is more of a mindset and decision-making tip.

Our bodies are made up of trillions of individual cells. Each one is like its own little universe. Very simply, disease is caused by only two things: toxicity or deficiency at the cellular level. Toxicity is too much of a bad thing. Deficiency is too little of a good thing.

Always keep in mind that anything you put in or on your body will affect your health on a cellular level. It will either move you toward sickness and disease, or toward health and wellness.

By staying hydrated, eating and using organic/natural products, periodic detoxifications, and sweating daily, you will be providing the cells in your body the optimal environment for health and wellness!

Remember, garbage in equals garbage out! If you put nasty products in or on your body, you'll get poor outcomes. If you fill your body with healthy, life-giving products, your body will respond with high levels of energy and performance!

MAXIMIZE NERVOUS SYSTEM FUNCTION

I believe this to be the most important key to your health! Why, you may ask? You can go weeks without food, days without water, minutes without oxygen, but you can't go one second without nerve supply!

Think about it…right now your heart is beating, lungs are breathing, intestines are digesting your last meal…and you don't even have to think about it! That's all being controlled by your nervous system.

The nervous system is made up of your brain, spinal cord, and the millions of nerves that come out from your spinal cord and branch out to all your organs, tissues, and cells. Think of it as a communication supernetwork within your body.

If there is any stress, irritation, or interference to the nervous system, it can affect the way your entire body functions and heals.

If you truly desire optimal health, it is crucial that you maintain a proper functioning nervous system throughout your entire life!

* CHIROPRACTIC CARE

As well as being a National Strength & Conditioning Association Certified Personal Trainer, I am a Doctor of Chiropractic. When you hear chiropractic, you might automatically think about neck or back pain. Chiropractic gets great results with neck and back pain, but what you might not know is that chiropractic also gets excellent results with conditions like:

- Headaches

- Difficulty Sleeping

- Numbness in Arms/Legs

- Sinus Problems

- Digestive Issues

- Whiplash Injuries

- Fatigue

- Lowered Immune Function

- Sciatica

- Carpal Tunnel Syndrome

- TMJ Disorder

- High/Low Blood Pressure

- Asthma

- Allergies

- Acid Reflux

- Scoliosis

- Ear Infections

- Colic

- Disc Herniations

- Vertigo

- Stress

- Vertebral Subluxation

Now, you might be thinking to yourself, "You chiropractors, you think you can cure everything!" If I had a dime for every time I heard that! The truth is, we don't cure ANYTHING! Nothing, zero, zilch, nada! Actually, no doctor in the world has ever cured anybody of anything. The ONLY person that can cure or heal anything is YOU (your own body)! That's it! A chiropractor's job is to simply get your body…all of your organs, tissues, and cells…FUNCTIONING optimally. When your body is functioning optimally, you have the very best chance to heal, whether it's a paper cut, cancer, or anything in between. Chiropractors work to increase your chances of living a long, happy life full of optimal health and radiant vitality!

You see, optimal health is NOT how you look or how you feel. There are plenty of people, celebrities, especially, that you can think of that looked fit and felt great, but were developing life-threatening diseases before any signs or symptoms were present. Please, do not judge your health by how you look or how you feel. Symptoms, or lack of symptoms, can be VERY misleading! 100% health = 100% function! It's how your body is functioning and healing that truly matters!

So, what controls the function and healing of all your organs, tissues, and cells? It's your nervous system! Your brain, spinal cord, and nerves.

Quick anatomy lesson for you…it doesn't matter if you're tall, short, heavy, thin, young, or old…you have the best doctor in the world, smarter than all doctors combined, right up in your brain. Your brain and nervous system transmit billions of nerve signals each and every second! Your brain sends messages down your spinal cord (at 270 mph), in through your nerves that come from your spinal cord, and out to all your organs, tissues, and cells. Also, the reverse happens… your organs, tissues, and cells send messages in through the nerves, up the spinal cord to the brain, telling it how they're doing and what they need.

Think of it as a safety pin. The top of the safety pin being your brain, the bottom being your body. As long as the safety pin is closed (connected), there can be a continuous loop of messages between the brain and body. The body can be at ease, functioning optimally.

Now, your brain is protected by your skull. Your spinal cord and nerve roots are protected by your spine…24 moveable bones (plus sacrum and coccyx) that provide structure and protection. If your spine is in the proper position, it is much stronger, but more importantly, the brain and body can communicate optimally.

However, due to the delicate relationship between the spine and the nervous system, when we have a shift in the spine, called a vertebral subluxation, it can cause stress, irritation or interference to the nervous system. This affects the messages between the brain and the body…think of the safety pin opened (disconnected). Now, the messages can't clearly, or at the optimal speed, get down and back up from the brain to the body, and from the body to the brain. This leads to dysfunction in the body, or dis-ease. Not disease, but dis-ease…lack of ease. Over time, that can lead to break down in any organ, tissue, or cell. The bad part is, this can be completely symptomless.

As chiropractors, we know two things:

1. Your body is the best doctor in the world. It can heal and repair itself. For example, let's say you cut your finger. If your body is functioning optimally, in a week or two, what will happen to that cut? Exactly…it heals!

2. For your body to function and heal optimally, you have to have optimal nerve supply. Another example… Let's say you go to your dentist. He or she slips and completely cuts a nerve to your tooth. What will happen to your tooth? Exactly…it will die. It doesn't matter how many times you brush it, floss it, or go back to the dentist, that tooth will die because there is no nerve supply, or life, getting to the tooth. Now, instead of completely cutting the nerve to your tooth, what would happen if your dentist somehow nicked, irritated, or pinched the nerve? Same thing…just to a lesser degree, right? So now, the tooth would probably start to turn colors, break down, and eventually, if left long enough without allowing the nerve to heal, cause a disease to the tooth. Make sense? So, here's the deal. Instead of that nerve going to your tooth, what if that irritated nerve was going to your heart, lungs, liver, kidney, thyroid, or digestive organs? Would you agree that those organs would not have the best chance to heal and repair themselves, and could eventually lead to break down? Yes! As chiropractors, our sole focus is to locate where there are shifts in the spine, which

causes stress, irritation or interference to the nervous system, and gently correct them through specific chiropractic adjustments.

Also, if your spine is out of alignment, it causes your spine, discs, and even your joints (feet, ankles, knees, hips, and shoulders) to wear out quicker. Just like if your car was out of alignment, your tires would wear out quicker.

Another comparison would be brushing your teeth. Why do you brush your teeth? To keep your teeth and gums healthy. Do you only brush your teeth when they hurt? Of course not. What would happen if you stopped brushing your teeth? Your teeth and gums would break down and cause problems. It's the exact same thing with your spine. Think about it…you can replace your teeth. I've yet to see a spinal transplant. If you neglect the health of your spine, it will break down and cause you health problems…far beyond just neck or back pain! The only reason chiropractors work on your neck and back is because that's where your "lifeline" (your spinal cord) is between your brain and your body. If it was down on your ankle…guess where we would be working more? Exactly!

Hippocrates, the father of modern medicine, stated, "Look well to the spine for the cause of disease!"

Thomas Jefferson was quoted as saying, "The doctor of the future will give no medicine, but will interest his patients in the care of the human frame (spine), in diet, and in the cause and prevention of disease."

Two very smart men, ahead of their time!

These spinal shifts, or vertebral subluxations, are caused by one thing…stress! Do you have any stress in your life? Don't worry, you're not alone! Now, there are three main types of stresses leading to vertebral subluxation that we call "The 3 T's": thoughts, toxins, and traumas.

Thoughts (Emotional Stress): finances, relationships, work, etc.

Toxins (Chemical Stress): the air we breathe, medications we take, what we eat, what we drink, what we put on our bodies, etc.

Traumas (Physical Stress): motor vehicle accidents, slips, falls, sports injuries, poor posture, poor sleeping habits, poor work ergonomics, the birthing process (for both mom and baby), etc.

The 3 T's can create a weakening and a shifting of the spine. To some degree, we all suffer from these stresses on a daily basis. This is why so many of my patients are astonished and upset when they look at their spinal x-rays for the first time. They ask, "Doc, how did my spine get in such bad shape?" It starts from day one, and it's a negative cumulative effect over years and years of stress.

So, what do your spinal x-rays look like? Do you know? When was the last time you had your spine and nervous system checked by a chiropractor? More importantly, what's the condition of your children's or grandchildren's spines?

Chiropractors are trained to locate and gently correct shifts (vertebral subluxations) in the spine. This will help your body to function at its very best, allowing you to do the things you love to do! Isn't that what we're all after?

This is why I choose to have my spine and nervous system checked by a chiropractor on a regular basis, and I encourage you to do the same.

POSTURE / ERGONOMICS

Posture is the window to the spine. If your posture is off, your spine is off. We have already discussed the negative health implications of spinal shifts.

One thing you need to do is to focus on having great posture whether you're standing, sitting, or sleeping. This will prevent degeneration of the spine, but also help supply your body with proper amounts of oxygen.

Try this quick posture experiment:

1. Stand or sit nice and tall with great ("proud") posture. Keep your chin up, pull your shoulders back, and hold your head back over your shoulders. Take a big, deep breath in through your nose, and notice how much oxygen you can take in. Quite a bit!

2. Now, stand or sit in slumped posture...shoulders rounded, head forward, with chin down slightly (as if you were slumped on the couch checking your text messages...seem familiar???). From this slumped posture, try to take another deep breath through your nose and notice how LITTLE oxygen you can take in. BIG difference, right?!

You're smart...do you think all your organs, tissues, cells, and muscles would benefit from more or less oxygen? You got it! More oxygen is a good thing, especially to prevent/battle cancer! Cancer cells HATE oxygen!

Focusing on your posture can improve your health neurologically, physiologically, and even emotionally (research shows that people who hold good posture are more confident, not the other way around). So, listen to your mother, and...."Sit/stand up straight!" ;)

When standing, pull your shoulders back, and keep your head back over your shoulders (instead of falling forward like when you're texting). We call it a proud posture.

When sitting, consider putting a pillow or lumbar support behind your lower back to maintain a healthy lumbar lordosis (curve). Also, try to keep computer screens at eye level or higher.

When sleeping, you basically have 3 options: back, side, or stomach.

Here are the pros and cons of each:

BACK:
 PROS:

- evenly distributes pressure on spine and discs

- allows for better circulation

 CONS:

- improper pillow causes stress on neck

- can increase snoring

SIDE:
 PROS:

- putting pillow between legs keeps pelvis level

- less snoring

- can help reduce acid reflux (left side specifically)

CONS:

- improper pillow causes stress on neck

- not alternating sides can cause strain on organs

STOMACH:
PROS:

- hardly any pros (less movement possibly)

CONS:

- reduces digestion and circulation

- neck strain from turning head one way or the other

- increases pressure on the lower back

- puts pressure on heart/lungs (using 25% more energy)

- may increase snoring/sleep apnea

My best recommendation would be to sleep on either your back or side and avoid stomach sleeping.

Personally, I try to sleep on my back or left side the majority of the time (with a pillow under or between my knees occasionally).

Also, no matter the position, make sure you have a pillow and a mattress that keep your body in a good posture. I recommend using as firm of a mattress/pillow you can handle. Everybody is different. Find out what works best for you.

SPINAL HYGIENE / CORE

The dental profession has done an amazing job educating people on the importance of preventative maintenance for dental health BEFORE problems occur. Because of this education and knowledge, we do things such as brush, floss, and visit our dentist on a regular basis. These activities have drastically reduced the number of dental health problems.

Why don't we take this same approach with our spines? Like I said earlier, we only get one spine; you can't replace it (like you can with teeth), and it has to last you your entire life.

80% of Americans will suffer from back or neck pain at some point, and the success rate for spinal surgeries is far from great. I'm confident that if we did some "spinal hygiene" on our own and visited the chiropractor on a regular basis, the amount of back pain, herniated/degenerated discs, and spinal surgeries would decrease drastically, much like the dental story!

Many of the debilitating spinal conditions that I see are caused by years of sedentary living or sitting a lot (i.e. desk jobs). Sitting to the spine is like candy to the teeth. It is essential to take the 24 moveable bones in our spine through healthy ranges of motion on a regular basis. This is why chiropractic care is so effective. Chiropractors find the bones in the spine that are stuck or not moving correctly and work to gently create proper motion. This allows the joint to avoid premature breakdown and degeneration…AKA degenerative disc disease.

Here are a few spinal hygiene movements that you can do at home, on a daily basis, which will help keep your spine healthy and functioning optimally!

* Please consult with your chiropractor/physician before

performing these exercises. If any pain or dizziness occurs, stop immediately and tell your doctor.

* Perform exercises on both sides of the body

* Continue to breathe while performing exercises

* Either perform 20-30 reps through a full range of motion OR hold for 20-30 seconds at a maximum range of motion

Neck Flexion – tuck your chin and gently flex your neck forward as far as possible

Neck Extension – extend head back as far as possible

Neck Rotation – turn head to one side as far as possible

Neck Lateral Flexion – side-bend your head, moving your ear toward your shoulder

Spinal Flexion – bend forward slowly, flexing the spine as if to touch your toes

Spinal Extension – place hands on hips and extend back, pointing chest to ceiling

Spinal Rotation – grasp hands together and rotate spine and head to one side

Spinal Lateral Flexion – bend to one side while sliding hand down the side of thigh

Think of this as "brushing and flossing" your spine. Your spine will thank you when you're able to play with your kids and grandkids without pain!

Also, I highly recommend you avoid performing a high volume of sit-ups, as they cause your spinal discs (shock absorbers between your spinal bones) to wear out quicker. I would much rather you do planks or bird dog exercises when training your core. These exercises provide strength and stability while protecting your spine from wear and tear.

VAGUS NERVE TONE

The vagus nerve is critical to optimal health. Vagus nerve means "wandering nerve" because it wanders all over the body and affects the function of many organs. It is part of the parasympathetic nervous system, or rest and digest system. The vagus nerve starts in the brainstem, just behind the ear, and connects the brain with organs such as the heart, stomach, intestines, liver, kidney, and lungs, just to name a few. It even affects your immune system.

Studies have shown that people with high vagus nerve tone have less inflammation, better organ function, better heart rate variability (an indicator of parasympathetic function), a stronger immune system, and overall better health.

So, how can we increase vagal tone naturally? Here are a few ways to do so (selfhacked.com):

- Cold water (showers or splashing face)

- Singing

- Humming

- Yoga

- Meditation

- Deep, slow breathes

- Laughter

- Prayer

- Exercise

- Probiotics

- Massage

- Fasting

- Sleep

- Tai Chi

- Chiropractic care

Increasing your vagal tone will help you prevent heart attack, stroke, depression, diabetes, and fatigue.

Chiropractors have been preaching the critical importance of brain, nerve, and body/organ connection since 1895. Modern medical research is just now catching up to what the chiropractic profession has been practicing for over 120 years!

Muscle Pliability

Tom Brady, the NFL superstar quarterback, has made muscle pliability a hot topic when he revealed his healthy lifestyle and training habits. He has stressed how important muscle pliability is to his performance and injury prevention.

Muscle pliability, according to Brady, can be defined as muscles that are lengthened, softened, and primed to fire properly. This will lead to optimal function and injury prevention when compared to tight, dense, and stiff muscles.

Whether you're a professional athlete or a stay-at-home mom, proper muscle pliability can help you perform at your best.

Several factors play a role in optimal muscle pliability:

- Diet: eating a plant-based, anti-inflammatory diet

- Hydration: drinking ½ your body weight in ounces of water per day

- Supplementation: omega-3s and electrolytes

- Strength Training: bodyweight and resistance band training

- Bodywork: pliability, massage, myofascial release, soft tissue work, muscle activation, foam rolling, chiropractic care, etc.

We were all born with natural muscle pliability, but it decreases as we get older. Think of how flexible and pliable a toddler is compared to the average 50-year-old. It is natural to lose some pliability, but our goal is to maintain it the best we can.

Through active pliability training, specifically contracting your muscles through movement, you can stimulate and re-educate your brain by creating new neural pathways.

I highly recommend you invest in a foam roller, and look to find a high-quality bodywork expert that will help you increase your muscle pliability to keep you performing at your best!

Remember, optimal function is the key to optimal health. I challenge you to pay close attention to the health of your spine, nervous system, muscles, and joints!

21-DAY OPTIMAL HEALTH CHALLENGE

Here's the truth; all the information in the world doesn't mean a thing if you don't take action. You can make or break a habit in just 21 days. I want to challenge you to put these health tips into play for the next 21 days, and notice how your life and health change!

Consult with your physician before starting any health program.

1) 4-7-8 BREATHING (2 MINUTES PER DAY)

- Inhale through the nose for 4, hold breath for 7, exhale through mouth for 8 (4-8x)

2) BURST TRAINING (2 MINUTES PER DAY)

- March, jog, or run in place as fast as you can for 3 x 20 ON/20 OFF

3) GREENS (6 MINUTES PER DAY)

- Eat one salad or drink a "greens" drink

4) WATER INTAKE (2 MINUTES PER DAY)

- Drink a large glass of water first thing in the morning

5) SPINE & NERVE SYSTEM ASSESSMENT (1 x 30 MINUTES)

- Schedule a spine and nerve system assessment with a quality chiropractor

* Total Time = 4 hours, 42 minutes

CONCLUSION

et me ask you…would you be excited to live to be 100 years old?

Whenever I ask that, some people are excited, but many people say, "No way, Doc!"

Those people that are not excited are typically picturing themselves at 100 years old, and they're thinking, "I won't have my health. I won't be able to do the things I love. I might be a burden to my family. I'd just rather not deal with it!"

Understandable, but let me reframe the question.

What if I had a crystal ball, and I could predict the future? I know who's going to win the Super Bowl. I know what the stock market is going to do. I also know that you are going to live to 100. No ifs, ands, or buts about it…you're living to 100! When do you think would be a good time to start getting healthy? 99? 98? Of course not! Today! Today is your day! Start taking action today. Procrastination is the thief of health! Start implementing the health tips in this book TODAY!

Here's the deal…the last thing I want is for you to finish reading this book and not take any action. I don't want that on my conscience. But more importantly, I don't want you to have to make your healthcare decisions from a hospital room or an emergency room.

Think about the last time you were in a hospital room or an emergency room. What did it look like? What did it sound like? What did it smell like? It's not exactly Disneyland, is it? Yet, I'm willing to bet that either you or somebody you know has had to make their healthcare decisions from a hospital room or an emergency room. They start health negotiations with God. "God, if you help me make it through this, I promise I'll start eating healthier! I promise I'll start exercising! I promise I'll quit smoking!"

The sad thing is, most of those good habits last about 90 days, and then they're right back into their old, bad habits!

Don't let that be you! Start taking action today! Make your health a priority now!

I'm in your corner and here for you 100%!

I know you can do it!

JOIN THE MISSION

"We never know how far reaching something we may think, say or do today will affect the lives of millions tomorrow." -B. J. Palmer

If you think this book has helped you in any way, we would be honored if you could share it with your friends and loved ones!

Also, if you could take two minutes and write a positive review on Amazon, it would be greatly appreciated!

You never know…by your generous gift or powerful words, you could change the life of someone that is looking to take their health to the next level!

I thank you in advance for joining the mission of helping people reach their full potential!

Best regards,

Dr. Chaz Ebert

FULL P⬤TENTIAL
CHIROPRACTIC

COMPLIMENTARY CHIROPRACTIC ASSESSMENT

If you're in the Athens/Oconee area, and looking to take your health to the next level, we would love to see if we can help you. Here at Full Potential Chiropractic, our mission is to help you live a happy and healthy life so you can do the things you love!

When you think about chiropractic, you probably think about neck pain and back pain. While we have helped thousands of people with neck pain and back pain, we have also helped people who suffer with many other health challenges, including:

- Fatigue
- Headaches
- Difficulty Sleeping
- Allergies
- Asthma
- Numbness in arms/legs
- Carpal Tunnel Syndrome
- Thyroid Dysfunction
- Digestive Problems
- Sciatica
- Dizziness
- TMJ Disorder
- High Blood Pressure
- Weak Immune System

Unfortunately, many people ignore their health, or worse yet, mask their symptoms while the underlying cause of the problem continues to progress. This typically leads to pain, sickness, disease, drugs, surgeries, high medical costs, and limited ability to live the life of your dreams. Our goal is to prevent these things by working to correct the true cause of your health challenges.

At this point you might be asking yourself: I wonder if chiropractic could help me? How long will it take to see results? How much will it cost? Will my insurance cover care? These are all great questions. That is why we offer all new patients a **Complimentary Chiropractic Assessment** to determine if the care we provide is right for you.

You will be able to sit down with Dr. Chaz Ebert; he will perform a personal consultation and a state-of-the-art neurological diagnostic test. At this point, Dr. Ebert will give you his best recommendations for you and your health before you incur any charges.

If you or a loved one is looking to take your health to the next level, all you need to do is give us a call at **706-403-2332** to schedule your Complimentary Chiropractic Assessment.

Here are just a few success stories from our practice members:

"I'm able to enjoy my children a lot more, and I feel like a different person!" – Nicole D.

"Dr. Ebert has changed my life. I'm not in constant pain anymore, and I enjoy my life again!" –Cheryl W.

"I haven't had a headache since my first adjustment. FPC has changed my life for the better!" – Allison J.

Call Today! We look forward to serving you!

Full Potential Chiropractic
2410 Hog Mountain Rd,
Watkinsville, GA 30677
706-403-2332
fpchiro.com

ABOUT THE AUTHOR

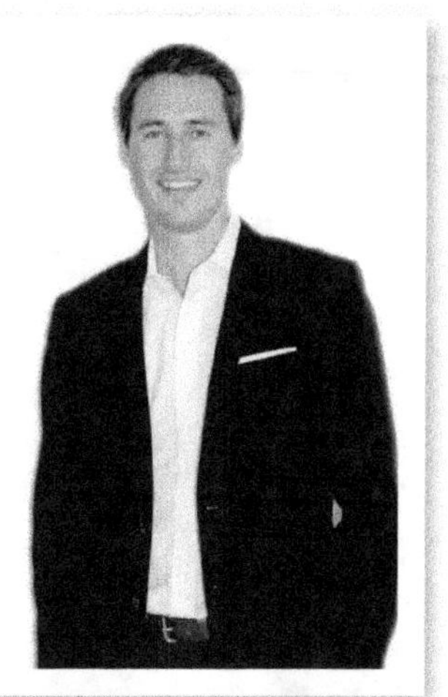

D r. Ebert is originally from Antigo, WI. He attended Murray State University in Murray, KY where he was an NCAA Division I First Team All-Conference baseball player. Dr. Ebert received his Doctorate of Chiropractic from Life University in Marietta, GA, where he graduated Cum Laude. He has also been a National Strength and Conditioning Association Certified Personal Trainer since 2006.

Dr. Ebert has spent the last 15+ years researching and studying the most advanced health and wellness principles in the world. He has traveled hundreds of thousands of miles and spent thousands of hours mastering these life-changing principles. Dr. Ebert has been featured in corporations, groups, and several radio shows throughout the country. He has been blessed to work with some of the largest wellness clinics in the world, helping people reach their full potential. Dr. Ebert has also done mission work in the Dominican Republic and homeless shelters.

When he is not in the office, Dr. Ebert enjoys playing golf, reading, music, and being on the lake. He is married to his wonderful wife, Lauren. They have a beautiful daughter, Anna.

ACKNOWLEDGMENTS

I have had so many wonderful mentors and resources to learn from over the years. I would like to thank: Dr. James Chestnut, Dr. Joseph Mercola, Dr. Josh Axe, Dr. Ben Lerner, Dr. Ted Smith, TB12 Method, and the National Strength & Conditioning Association.

I would also like to thank my beautiful wife, Lauren, for all her love and support. I love you more than ever, Babe! You and Anna are my everything!

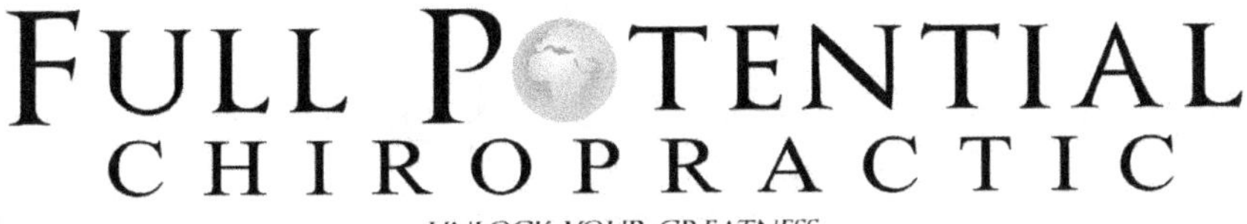

2410 HOG MOUNTAIN ROAD

WATKINSVILLE, GA 30677

706-403-2332

FPCHIRO.COM